# ESSENTIAL GUIDE TO SCABIES

## Comprehensive Insights for Effective Management and Recovery

**DR. CASEY LOREN**

# DISCLAIMER

This book's content is only meant to be used for general informative purposes. Although the author has taken great care to ensure the content is accurate and thorough, no warranties or assurances on the information's accuracy, correctness, or reliability are provided. It is recommended that readers employ their own judgment and discretion when applying any material found in this book to their particular situation.

The information in this book is not intended to replace professional advice, nor is the author an expert in any of the subjects covered. It is recommended that readers consult with experienced professionals regarding any particular issues or concerns.

Any name that may be mentioned or referred in this book does not imply endorsement, recommendation, or relationship on the part of the author with any person, entity, good, website, or association. These references are made only for informational purposes and are not meant to be taken as recommendations or endorsements.

The information contained in this book may cause readers to suffer loss or damage, for which the author disclaims all obligation and accountability. The only people accountable for the decisions and actions taken by readers using the information presented are themselves.

Any names, characters, companies, locations, activities, occasions, and incidents referenced in this book are either made up or the result of the author's imagination. Any likeness to real people, living or dead, or to real things is entirely coincidental.

This book's content may change at any time, without prior notice, according to the author. The onus is on the reader to verify whether there have been any updates or revisions.

The reader accepts the conditions of this disclaimer by reading this book. Please do not read this book or use its contents if you do not agree to these terms.

**Table of Contents**

# CHAPTER 1
## GETTING TO KNOW SCABIES

### How Scabies Are Defined:

The small mite Sarcoptes scabiei is the infectious agent responsible for scabies, a skin infestation. These tiny mites cause a rash that looks like pimples and severe itching when they burrow into the skin. Close physical contact is all it takes for scabies to spread from person to person.

### Present and Past

At least two accounts of scabies have been found in ancient texts, one each from Greece and Rome. In the 17th century, the Italian physician Giovanni Cosimo Bonomo was the first to identify the mite that causes scabies. Much progress has been made in the medical field's comprehension and treatment of scabies since then.

# What makes scabies ticks

The skin is the sole host for the Sarcoptes scabies mite, the causative agent of scabies. Itching and a rash are symptoms of an allergic reaction caused by mites that burrow into the skin to lay eggs. Most cases of scabies spread from person to person through long periods of skin-to-skin contact.

# Indications & Warning Flags

Severe itching, particularly at night, a rash resembling a pimple, tiny holes or tracks in the skin, and wounds brought on by scratching are common indications of scabies. In most cases, the rash will manifest in crevices or folds, like the spaces between the fingers, the wrists, the elbows, the knees, and the genitalia.

# Scabies Diagnosis

Scabies are usually diagnosed by physically examining the skin for telltale characteristics like burrows, rash, and blisters. Under a microscope, mites, eggs, or feces can be identified from skin scrapings or biopsies.

## Scabies Transmission

Prolonged, skin-to-skin contact with an infected individual is the main vector for the transmission of scabies. Beds, clothes, and furnishings that are infected can potentially spread the disease indirectly. The risk of transmission is increased for those who are sexually or domestically intimate.

## Elements of Danger

People with compromised immune systems, those who live in close quarters with infected people, those who share clothing or bedding, and those who live in crowded or institutional environments are more likely to have scabies. Those most at risk are the young, the old, and those with weak immune systems.

## It gets more complicated

Scabies, if untreated, can cause impetigo, a nasty and infectious skin infection, crusted scabies, and post-scabies itch, which is an itchy skin condition that doesn't go away even after therapy. Skin injury and subsequent infections are additional risks associated with scratching.

## Common False Beliefs

Scabies is often believed to be a sexually transmitted disease or that it just affects those with bad hygiene, among other false beliefs. Although it is most commonly transmitted through intimate physical contact, scabies can infect anyone.

## Taking Steps to Avoid Problems:

Scabies prevention measures include not sharing personal belongings, washing bedding and clothing frequently, and avoiding intimate contact with infected people. To stop the spread of the infection, infected people and those who come into touch with them must be treated quickly.

# CHAPTER 2

## SCABIES MITE ANATOMY

## Scabies mites are described as follows:

Microscopic parasites known as scabies mites (Sarcoptes scabiei) infest the skin of some animals and humans. Along with ticks and spiders, they are members of the arachnid family. You can hardly see these mites because they are translucent and only approximately 0.3 to 0.4 millimeters long. In addition to having four pairs of legs, which enable them to hop from one piece of skin to another, their bodies are oval.

## A Scabies Mite's Life Cycle:

Scabies mites go through several phases in their life cycle. Following mating on the skin's surface, the female mite will dig a hole in the epidermis to deposit her eggs. The life cycle of a mite begins with an egg and continues with its larvae, nymphs, and adulthood. It usually takes about two to four weeks for the entire life cycle to complete. This is when the mites gorge themselves on dead skin, bodily fluids, and other tissue remnants.

## How Scabies Mites Are Structured

The unique anatomy of scabies mites allows them to live and multiply within their host. Fine hairs and spines cover their body, allowing them to move around and cling to the skin. In addition, they have specialized mouthparts that allow them to penetrate flesh and draw out nutrients. To further aid in their feeding process, mites release enzymes that aid in the breakdown of skin proteins.

## Actions and Routines

The scabies mite is primarily active at night because it is a nocturnal animal. To ensure their survival and procreation, they seek out habitats that are warm and damp. These mites are extremely infectious and can spread from person to person just by being physically close to an infected person. Additionally, they can temporarily live on non-host materials like clothing, bedding, or furniture.

## Places Where Insects Occur

Infestations of scabies mites are widespread in locations with thin or folded skin, such as the interdigital spaces, the insides of the fingers and wrists, the armpits, the waistline, the buttocks, and the vaginal area. On the other hand, they aren't limited to just those areas; the scalp, face, hands, and feet are all fair game. The burrowing and feeding activities of the mites cause severe itching, which is a hallmark symptom of scabies, especially at night.

## Adjustments for the Senses

Scabies mites can find hosts by utilizing sensory modifications that allow them to navigate their environment. Legs and bodies equipped with sensory organs let them pick up on temperature changes, chemical signals, and other signs from their surroundings. Mites have adapted so that they can find the best parts of the skin to feed and multiply in.

## How We Stay Alive

To stay alive, scabies mites use a variety of strategies, both on their hosts and off. Being concealed in clothes, bedding, or furniture allows them to live for multiple days without a host. Their capacity to burrow into the epidermis also shields them from predators and enables them to feed and procreate even when the host body's immune system reacts negatively.

## Methods for Having Children

For the sake of their survival and proliferation, scabies mites reproduce at a high pace. There can be a dramatic spike in the population of mites very quickly since females can lay eggs numerous times a day. Scabies infections can last for a long time and spread easily in crowded or dirty places because of how efficiently they reproduce.

# Interaction with the Host

The parasitic disease scabies is caused by the tight relationship between human hosts and scabies mites. A variety of symptoms, such as itching, skin rash, and even secondary bacterial infections, are caused by this interaction. Inflammation and the development of telltale skin burrows and nodules are outcomes of the immunological response that the mites elicit in their hosts.

# Problems with Treatmen

The mites' capacity to live independently of the host and their high reproductive rate present multiple obstacles to controlling scabies infestations. Topical treatments like permethrin or oral medications like ivermectin are commonly used to treat mites and their eggs. It is important to treat all infected patients and their close contacts at the same time to avoid treatment failure or reinfestation. Treatment attempts can be further complicated in some circumstances when particular drugs develop resistance.

To effectively manage and prevent infestations, it is necessary to understand the anatomy, life cycle, behavior, and treatment problems of scabies mites.

# CHAPTER 3

## EPIDEMIOLOGY OF SCABIES

## Worldwide Rates of Incidence

The skin condition known as scabies is caused by the Sarcoptes scabies mite, which is extremely contagious. Regional and population factors significantly affect global incidence rates. The incidence rates are typically greater in resource-poor places, have overpopulation, and have inadequate access to healthcare. But scabies are still an issue, especially in institutionalized places like jails and nursing homes, even in industrialized nations.

## Patterns of Demographics

Scabies has little respect for gender, age, or socioeconomic level; it can strike anyone. Nonetheless, specific demographic tendencies emerge. Close quarters in homes and schools make children more susceptible to scabies, which is especially common in areas with poor incomes. Occupational exposure, especially for people in the healthcare or caregiving industries, can raise the risk.

## Seasonal patterns

In some places, the incidence of scabies varies with the seasons. Cases may be at their highest in temperate regions during the winter when individuals tend to stay indoors more. Seasonal patterns may be less noticeable in tropical regions, on the other hand, due to the consistently pleasant weather.

## Location-Based Distribution

The spread of scabies is not constant, yet it is present on a global scale. Because mites thrive in warm, humid environments, their incidence tends to be higher in tropical and subtropical locations. Though affluent nations with good healthcare systems are not immune to outbreaks, they can happen anywhere.

## Groups and Outbreaks

Healthcare institutions, educational institutions, and refugee camps are among the places where scabies outbreaks have been known to occur. Clusters of instances are caused by the transmission of mites through close contact. The key to controlling outbreaks and stopping their spread is quick diagnosis, treatment, and prevention.

## Impact on Public Health

Particularly for at-risk communities, scabies pose serious public health concerns. Social stigma, additional bacterial infections, and severe itching are all possible outcomes. Scabies can cause issues and higher healthcare expenditures in places like nursing homes or with people who have impaired immune systems.

# Economic and Social Considerations

The epidemiology of scabies is influenced by socioeconomic factors. Greater prevalence rates are found in underprivileged communities because of factors such as poverty, overcrowding, inadequate sanitation, and restricted access to healthcare. Controlling and preventing scabies effectively requires addressing these variables.

# Impacts on the Environment

The transmission of scabies can be influenced by environmental factors such as weather, housing, and personal cleanliness habits. Mites transmit from person to person by skin-to-skin contact and flourish in damp, warm climates. Reducing transmission risk can be achieved through enhancing living circumstances and promoting hygiene education.

# New Problems

Drug resistance and the effects of migration are new concerns in the field of scabies epidemiology. It is important to develop alternate treatments and monitoring programs because scabicide resistance is a major worry. It is necessary to coordinate monitoring and control activities since migration patterns also contribute to the global spread of scabies.

# Methods for Control

Combinations of measures are necessary for effective scabies control tactics. Early diagnosis, scabicide treatment, contact tracing, sanitation education, and targeted interventions in high-risk areas are all part of the plan. The success of control programs depends on community involvement and cooperation among healthcare practitioners, public health organizations, and communities themselves.

To reduce transmission, improve public health outcomes, and implement targeted interventions, it is essential to understand the epidemiology of scabies. To overcome the obstacles presented by this skin invasion, continuous study, monitoring, and cooperation are essential.

# CHAPTER 4

## SCABIES SYMPTOMS IN THE CLINIC

### Traditional Scabies

The usual appearance of a scabies infection is known as classic scabies. When you get a severe case of nighttime itching, it's because your body is reacting allergically to mites, their eggs, and their excrement. The most common sign is the presence of tiny, wavy lines on the skin—burrows—that can be any color and can be seen between the fingers, on the wrists, elbows, armpits, waist, genitalia, and buttocks. Scratching can lead to secondary infections of the skin, little red lumps, and rashes that resemble pimples are other common symptoms.

### The Norwegian Scabies Crusted

Norwegian scabies, or crusted scabies, is an extremely infectious and painful kind of scabies.

An abundance of mites and their eggs is contained within a thick layer of skin that is characteristic of this condition. Crusty scabies, in contrast to classic scabies, might produce mild desensitization of the skin rather than severe itching at first. You might notice the crusts on your hands, feet, elbows, knees, and even your scalp. Immunocompromised people, the elderly, and people with neurological disorders are at increased risk for this scabies kind.

## Unusual Displays

It can be tough to diagnose scabies since it can occasionally manifest in unusual ways. Nodular scabies, bullous scabies, scabies incognito, and scalp involvement are examples of atypical presentations. Nodules instead of burrows, big blisters, and a changed look after topical steroids are all possible. Not being conversant with these variances can cause healthcare providers to delay diagnosis and treatment.

## Possible Diagnosis

Other skin illnesses like eczema, dermatitis, insect bites, and fungal infections can also cause itching and skin lesions, which might lead to a differential diagnosis of scabies. To treat and manage scabies effectively, it is essential to distinguish them from these disorders.

## Problems and Their Consequences

As a result of the itching and open wounds caused by scabies, secondary bacterial infections such as impetigo and cellulitis can develop. It is possible to develop systemic infections in extreme situations, particularly with crusted scabies. Psychosocial impacts, sleep disruptions, and a diminished quality of life are additional outcomes of scabies infestations.

## Child SafetyThings to Think About

Scabies affect children frequently because of the tight quarters they experience in places like schools and daycares. Lesions on the cheeks, palms, and soles are among the areas where infants could show symptoms. To stop the disease from spreading and causing difficulties, it is crucial to treat scabies in youngsters as soon as possible.

## Factors to Consider for the Elderly

Crumbly scabies are more common in the elderly because of immune system alterations brought on by aging and other diseases. Scabies in the elderly might manifest in unusual ways, which can cause diagnostic delays and treatment delays. Healthcare providers and carers should be extra careful while diagnosing and treating scabies in this group.

## Patients with Reduced Immune Function

Severe and unusual scabies infections are more common in immunocompromised people, including those who have HIV/AIDS, have received an organ transplant, or are taking immunosuppressive medication. The high mite burden and risk of complications make crusted scabies particularly common and tough to control in this patient group.

## Socio-Emotional Impacts

Anxiety, despair, social stigma, and a diminished quality of life are some of the serious psychological impacts that people may experience as a result of a scabies infestation. Experiencing scabies can be emotionally taxing and disruptive to daily life and relationships due to the itching, visible skin lesions, and contagiousness of the disease.

## Impact on Quality of Life

Scabies hurt people's lives that go beyond only the physical symptoms. It has the potential to impact one's mental health, social life, ability to sleep, and attendance at work or school. Treatment of the infestation is only part of effective scabies care; patients also need emotional support to help them cope with the disease and lead better lives.

Early detection, correct diagnosis, and holistic treatment are crucial for minimizing problems and improving results; this thorough guide covers the clinical manifestations of scabies across different groups and presentations.

# CHAPTER 5
## HOW TO DIAGNOSE SCABIES

### Clinical Evaluation

Medical professionals take a patient's symptoms, medical history, and the results of a physical exam into account when diagnosing scabies. The development of tiny, raised bumps or blisters and severe itching, particularly at night, are key signs. Finding secondary skin alterations, such as excoriations from scratching, and distinctive skin lesions, including burrows and nodules, are also part of the clinical evaluation.

### Methods for Examining the Skin

Scabies skin exams include looking closely at the afflicted regions, such as folds of skin, genitalia, and crevices between the fingers, and wrists. When you look closely enough using a dermatoscope or magnifying glass, you can see the mites' distinctive sores and burrows—tiny, thread-like patterns in the skin.

## Results from Dermoscopy

Scabies can be diagnosed with dermoscopy, which can show particular features such as linear tunnels, mite parts, and inflammatory changes. The mite's burrow is represented by a center black dot and appears as delicate, wavy brown lines. Symptoms of inflammation include redness, scaling, and the development of tiny papules.

## Laboratory Evaluations

The presence of mites, eggs, or fecal pellets can be determined through microscopic examination of skin scrapings, which are part of the laboratory testing process for scabies. Additionally, scabies DNA can be detected by polymerase chain reaction (PCR) assays. The results of these tests might not be required for a diagnosis in cases where the clinical evidence is sufficient.

## Possible Diagnosis

Insect bites, eczema, and contact dermatitis are just a few of the skin disorders that scabies can resemble. By comparing symptoms, medical history, and, in some cases, laboratory results, a differential diagnosis can be made to rule out other, seemingly related disorders.

## Problems with Diagnosis

Scabies have symptoms with various skin diseases and can manifest in a variety of ways, making a diagnosis difficult. Delays or missed diagnoses might occur when symptoms are unusual or when subsequent infections obscure them.

## Dependability and Precision

Scabies diagnosis relies on a mix of clinical evaluation, skin examination methods, and occasionally laboratory testing to ensure accuracy and dependability. The diagnostic accuracy of scabies lesions is typically higher when performed by clinicians who have familiarity with them.

## Programs for Screening

In densely populated areas, healthcare facilities, nursing homes, and other high-risk groups, scabies screening programs are necessary. Scabies prevention programs include skin exams regularly, education on the subject, and rapid treatment of instances found to stop the spread of the disease.

## Uses of Telemedicine

Scabies diagnosis using telemedicine is on the rise, particularly in underserved areas or during pandemics when access to in-person consultations is at a premium. Scabies can be more accurately diagnosed and treated with the help of virtual consultations, patient-provided pictures, and medical history.

## What's to Come

New point-of-care testing for scabies, including quick antigen detection kits or diagnostic apps for smartphones, might be developed in the future. Potentially improving diagnostic accuracy and streamlining management methods are developments in AI and imaging technology.

Healthcare providers can improve patient outcomes and decrease disease burden by thoroughly knowing and using these components to diagnose and manage scabies.

# CHAPTER 6

## OPTIONS FOR TREATING SCABIES

## Scabicides for the Skin

The primary method of treating scabies involves the use of topical scabicides, which are administered directly to the skin to eliminate the mites and their eggs. Permethrin, crotamiton, and benzyl benzoate are some of the most often utilized topical agents. Applying permethrin from the neck down and rinsing it off after a set amount of time—typically 8–14 hours—is the most effective and recommended method. Other choices include crotamiton and benzyl benzoate, however, these may be less efficient and necessitate more applications. Careful adherence to the directions is required for optimal application and results.

# Medication Taken Orally

Oral drugs, such as ivermectin, may be recommended when topical therapies fail or are not feasible. Outbreaks or widespread scabies infestations are the best times to utilize ivermectin. The mites are paralyzed and killed by it. A healthcare expert should be responsible for managing the dosage and administration of oral medications because of the risk of side effects and combinations with other drugs.

# Alternate Methods of Treatment

A relaxing bath with oatmeal or baking soda added can help ease the itching and discomfort caused by scabies, as can other complementary therapies. It is important to note that these therapies should be taken with prescribed pharmaceuticals and should not be utilized in place of medical treatment.

# Possible Substitute Therapies

Ointments containing sulfur, tea tree oil, or neem oil are among the alternative treatments that are frequently recommended. There is limited scientific evidence to support the use of these in treating scabies, however, there may be anecdotal evidence of their efficacy. Alternative treatments might not be as safe or successful as traditional ones, so it's important to talk to a doctor before trying them.

# Treatment Recommendations

As a general rule, topical scabicides are the gold standard for treating scabies, with oral treatments being reserved for extreme cases. To avoid reinfestation, it is crucial to treat all household members and close contacts at the same time, according to the guidelines.

# Problems with Resistance

Scabies mites can become resistant to some treatments with time, especially if they are overused or mistreated. To tailor treatment plans to specific areas, healthcare practitioners should monitor resistance trends. In instances of resistance, it may be essential to employ combination therapy or consider alternate drugs.

# Potential Side Effects

Scabies treatments can cause some people to experience minor and transitory side effects. Redness, itching, or irritation of the skin are possible side effects. Though they are uncommon, people should contact their doctor right once if they experience a severe allergic response.

# Regimes for Treatment

The choice of medicine and the severity of the infestation determine the scabies treatment schedule. These treatments typically include a mix of oral and topical drugs or numerous applications of a topical scabicide. To assess the efficacy of treatment and deal with any persistent symptoms, follow-up exams are crucial.

## Care After the Fact

To determine whether the scabies treatment was successful and to deal with any residual symptoms or reinfestation, it is essential to undergo follow-up care. Proper hygiene habits, such as washing clothes and bedding in hot water and vacuuming furniture to get rid of any leftover mites or eggs, should be recommended to patients.

## Educating Patients

Effective management of scabies relies on patient education regarding the disease, its transmission, treatment choices, and preventative strategies.

Patients should know that it's crucial to finish their medication as prescribed, stay away from people until their doctor gives the all-clear, and tell those close to them to be checked out if they need to. Comprehensive care and support for patients coping with scabies is ensured through regular follow-up sessions and discussions with healthcare experts.

# CHAPTER 7

## CONTROLLING INFESTATIONS OF SCABIES

## Managing Your Home

Scabies prevention measures are an important part of home management. Things like:

1. **Identification and Diagnosis:** Being able to identify scabies by looking for symptoms like severe itching and skin rashes, and then immediately seeking medical help for a diagnosis.

2. **Treatment of Infested Individuals:** Treating all susceptible members of the household with the proper scabies medication, which is usually a topical lotion or cream containing permethrin or ivermectin.

3. To lessen the likelihood of reinfestation, it is important to practice good hygiene by taking baths regularly, washing linens, clothing, and towels in hot water, and keeping a clean living space.

4. To stop the spread of the disease, it is recommended that affected people stay away from other people in the house who are not sick until treatment is finished.

## Setting in Institutions

When dealing with scabies in institutional settings such as schools, nursing homes, or prisons, there are additional factors to consider:

1. **Screening Programmes:** Establishing regular screenings to identify scabies patients beforehand and forestall epidemics.

2. **Isolation and Treatment:** Controlling the infestation requires isolating those who are sick, treating them, and making sure they follow all necessary hygiene protocols.

3. **Awareness and Education:** Raising knowledge among employees, residents, and visitors regarding scabies symptoms, ways to prevent it, and the significance of following treatment instructions.

# Strategies for the Community

To control scabies in bigger populations, community-wide methods are essential:

1. Educating the public about scabies, how they spread, and available treatment options is the goal of **education campaigns**.

2. Working together with healthcare providers to speed up diagnosis, treatment, and follow-up for those impacted by the disease.

3. The use of environmental cleanliness measures in public areas to lessen the likelihood of scabies transmission is an example of an environmental measure.

# Training for Health Workers

Effective scabies management requires health staff to undergo proper training:

1. Healthcare personnel should be trained to correctly identify scabies using microscopic examination of skin scrapings and clinical presentation.

2. **Treatment procedures:** Making sure that medical staff understand the suggested treatment procedures, which include dosing, administration, and follow-up treatment.

3. **Patient Education:** Teaching medical professionals how to effectively communicate with patients to reduce the spread of scabies, encourage treatment compliance, and outline ways to avoid the disease.

## Systems for Monitoring

Robust monitoring systems can be set up to keep an eye on scabies outbreaks and trends:

1. **Case Reporting:** Establishing systems whereby healthcare providers can notify public health authorities of scabies instances to facilitate monitoring and response.

2. **Data Analysis:** Tracking scabies prevalence trends, high-risk populations, and geographic hotspots through the examination of surveillance data.

3. *Early Warning Systems:** Creating methods to identify and react quickly to spikes in scabies cases or epidemics.

# Adherence to the Treatment Plan

For scabies treatment to be effective, it is essential that affected individuals follow their treatment plan:

1. **Information and Guidance:** Informing patients and their caretakers of the significance of finishing the entire scabies treatment regimen through the provision of precise instructions, educational materials, and counseling.

2. **Follow-Up Care:** Planning follow-up visits to check in on how treatment is going, handle any

issues or side effects, and make sure everyone is sticking to their treatment plan.

3. **Support Services:** Assisting patients with their treatment regimen adherence by providing support services like transportation assistance or reminders.

## Locating a Contact

The goal of contact tracing is to find people who could have been exposed to scabies so that they might be treated:

1. **Case Investigations:** Carers, family members, and anybody else who had close skin-to-skin contact with a confirmed case of scabies should be located through comprehensive investigations.

2. To stop the spread of the disease and any future outbreaks, it is necessary to screen and treat those who have been identified as contacts.

3. Educating contacts about scabies, their symptoms, and how to avoid getting infected is an important part of preventing the disease.

## Controlling Outbreaks

To manage scabies epidemics, swift and coordinated interventions are essential:

1. **Rapid Response Teams:** forming groups to act swiftly in response to scabies epidemics in hospitals, schools, and other places.

2. To control the spread of the disease, it is necessary to establish isolation sites and provide accelerated treatment for those who need it.

3. Healthcare providers, public health organizations, and impacted institutions can work together more efficiently to execute control measures if they can communicate and coordinate with one another.

# Partnerships and Collaborations

To effectively control scabies, collaboration, and collaborations are crucial:

1. Healthcare, education, social services, and community organizations are all part of the multi-sectoral collaboration that aims to tackle scabies from many perspectives.

2. Working together with private healthcare providers, pharmaceutical companies, and non-governmental organizations to enhance access to diagnostic, treatment, and prevention services is known as a **public-private partnership**.

3. Strengthening scabies control efforts globally requires international cooperation, which includes taking part in global initiatives and exchanging best practices with other nations.

# Important Takeaways

Strategies for controlling scabies in the future can be informed by thinking back on what has worked and what hasn't:

1. **Epidemic Preparedness:** Creating and honing plans for handling epidemics to improve response capabilities by learning from previous outbreaks.

2. To effectively control scabies, it is crucial to include the community, create trust, and use culturally sensitive approaches.

3. The improvement of scabies diagnosis, treatment choices, and preventative measures can be achieved by investments in research and innovation.

Communities can control scabies infestations successfully and limit their impact on public health by addressing these areas comprehensively and collectively.

# CHAPTER 8

## Scabs and the Welfare of the Public

### Illness Burden

The skin condition known as scabies is caused by the Sarcoptes scabies mite, which is extremely contagious. An estimated 200 million instances are recorded every year, affecting people from all walks of life and all walks of age. Scabies is a hardship in and of itself, but they also causes social shame and lowers the quality of life on top of the physical pain. Overcrowding and a lack of resources make it more common in places like elderly homes and refugee camps.

### Effect on the Economy:

Direct healthcare costs, lost productivity from sickness, and expenses linked to managing outbreaks in institutions all contribute to the enormous economic effect of scabies. Healthcare systems and individuals in low-income areas may struggle to afford the treatment of scabies and its consequences, such as secondary bacterial infections, due to a lack of healthcare resources.

## A Framework for Policy

To effectively combat scabies, strong policy frameworks are required. This encompasses protocols for monitoring and controlling outbreaks in addition to standards for diagnosis, treatment, and prevention. Prioritizing vulnerable populations and fostering collaboration among healthcare providers, government agencies, and community organizations should also be part of policy initiatives.

## To promote health equity

Resolving socioeconomic determinants of health, including poverty, overcrowding, and insufficient healthcare access, is essential for attaining health equity in scabies prevention and management. Everyone, regardless of their financial situation or where they live, should be able to affordably and easily get scabies treatment and preventive alternatives.

## Systems for Surveillance:

Monitoring the prevalence of scabies, identifying outbreaks, and evaluating the impact of management efforts all require robust surveillance systems. Regular data collecting, reporting systems, and cooperation between healthcare providers and public health officials are all part of this process, which allows for the monitoring of trends and the application of appropriate targeted interventions.

## Strategies for Intervention:

Mass drug administration (MDA) in high-prevalence areas, targeted treatment of afflicted people and close contacts, health education and promotion, and environmental measures to prevent mite transmission are all part of the scabies intervention strategy. To put these plans into action, healthcare providers, community organizers, and public health specialists must work together as interdisciplinary teams.

## Missions to Raise Awareness:

To encourage early diagnosis, treatment-seeking behaviorbehavior, and preventive actions against scabies, public awareness campaigns are crucial. Campaigns like these should educate people about scabies symptoms, debunk common misconceptions, and promote cleanliness in the home and community as a a means to cut down on mite transmission.

## Main Areas of Study:

Improving early detection diagnostic tools, creating new treatment modalities, studying scabies epidemiology in various populations, determining the effect of interventions on disease burden, and studying the host immune response in scabies pathogenesis are all important areas of focus for scabies research. To successfully address these priorities, research collaborations between academic institutions, businesses, and government agencies are required.

## Worldwide Projects:

Coordinating worldwide efforts to prevent scabies requires global actions. Mobilizing resources, advocating for policy changes, and supporting research and implementation initiatives in high-burden regions are all goals of partnerships between international organizations, governments, philanthropic foundations, and non-governmental organizations (NGOs).

## Aims for Advocacy:

The neglected tropical disease of scabies must be brought to the attention of the public through advocacy efforts if we are to see it adequately funded, resourced, and politically committed to ending its spread. As part of larger global health initiatives, advocates may mobilize the public, impacted communities, healthcare practitioners, and lawmakers to make scabies management and prevention a top priority.

Public health initiatives can greatly alleviate scabies and improve health outcomes for communities and individuals afflicted by tackling all of these factors simultaneously.

# CHAPTER 9

## SCIENTIFIC PROGRESS ON SCABIES

### Research on Mite Biology

Researchers have taken a keen interest in mite biology due to the prevalence of scabies, which is caused by the Sarcoptes scabies mite. The life cycle, reproduction, and interactions of the mite with the skin of its hosts are all areas that researchers investigate. The development of more precise interventions to interrupt mite life cycles and decrease transmission can be facilitated by a better understanding of their biology.

### • Interactions between hosts and parasites

The complex interplay between the host and parasite is central to the study of scabies. A better understanding of the disease's mechanics can be achieved by investigating how Sarcoptes scabiei interacts with human skin, avoids immune responses, and causes itching and lesions. New vaccines and treatment approaches are based on what is known about the host-parasite interaction.

## Important Findings in Immunology

New information about the complicated immune responses caused by the Sarcoptes scabies infestation has emerged from the field of scabies study. To create more effective vaccines and therapeutic strategies for modifying immune reactivity, it is necessary to understand the immunological pathways that are involved in protective and pathogenic responses.

## Genetic Studies

Scabies vulnerability, host defenses, and mite virulence factors can be better understood by genetic investigations. Genomic studies have opened the door to targeted interventions and personalized medicine by revealing genetic variants that affect the severity of disease and the efficacy of treatments.

## Innovations in Treatment

New topical medicines, oral therapy, and combinations of current medications are examples of innovative techniques for treating scabies. Emerging drug resistance, safety, and effectiveness are the main areas of research. Alternative treatments, such as natural chemicals, and innovative medication delivery technologies show potential in scabies management.

## Diagnostic Tools

Modern diagnostic tools have completely altered the scabies detection and tracking processes. Rapid and precise diagnosis improves patient care and epidemiological monitoring, and it can be achieved using a variety of methods, including conventional skin scrapings, new imaging techniques, and molecular testing.

## Models for Epidemiology

Epidemiological models provide light on the dynamics of scabies transmission, risk factors, and the prediction of outbreaks. Effective scabies management can be aided by mathematical modeling in our understanding of disease propagation, evaluation of control techniques, and formulation of public health policy.

## Approaches to Monitoring

Digital health technologies, electronic medical records, and population-based surveys are some of the sophisticated surveillance methods that have been found to improve scabies monitoring and reporting. Improving disease surveillance, enabling early intervention, and tracking treatment outcomes are all made possible with real-time data collecting.

## Initiatives to Improve Public Health

Integrated healthcare treatments, community education, and hygiene promotion are all part of public health interventions for scabies. Scabies control and preventive efforts rely heavily on contact tracing programs, mass drug administration campaigns, and targeted treatments in areas with a high prevalence of the disease.

## Looking Ahead

Numerous promising avenues for scabies research in the future have been identified. Some of these areas of focus include developing better vaccines, finding new ways to treat scabies, using technology to improve telemedicine and remote patient monitoring, and working together on a global scale to combat the disease. To drive innovation and improve disease management internationally, it is important to embrace transdisciplinary approaches and engage stakeholders.

# CHAPTER 10

## MANAGING SCABIES

### How to Deal with Stress

Both the physical and mental tolls of scabies can be hard to bear. To cope, one must find ways to deal with the emotional fallout as well as the physical symptoms. Some examples of this include being very conscientious about taking all of your medication as directed, keeping up with your personal hygiene routine, and reaching out to people you care about for emotional support. To help manage the illness, it can be helpful to find ways to relax and minimize stress.

### Help for the Mind

The emotional and psychological toll of scabies treatment is real. Therapy sessions with mental health experts, support groups, or even just chatting freely with loved ones about how you're feeling and what you're worried about are all great ways to get psychological support. When problems with worry, sadness, or other emotions emerge, it is critical to deal with them.

## Changes to One's Way of Life

Changes to regular practices and behaviors are typically necessary for people living with scabies. Some of these measures include keeping personal hygiene up to par, cleaning clothes and bedding often, and limiting contact with other people while you're being treated. For scabies treatment to be effective, it is essential to follow certain lifestyle changes.

## Family relationships

Scabies is a family disease that can impact more than just one person. Family members affected by the problem must be encouraged to talk openly about it, adhere to treatment plans, and take precautions to stop the infestation from spreading. Dealing with scabies requires understanding and assistance from loved ones.

## Affective Discrimination

Misconceptions regarding the etiology and transmission of scabies might contribute to the social stigma that the disease can evoke. Reducing stigma and increasing understanding can be achieved by self- and community education regarding the disease. Overcoming the social stigma associated with scabies requires open communication and empathy from friends, colleagues, and communities.

## Resources for Help

When dealing with scabies, it can be quite helpful to build a support system. Healthcare providers, support organizations, internet forums, or reliable friends and family members can all be part of this network and provide invaluable insight, perspective, and comfort. One of the most important things you can do to help yourself cope with scabies is to surround yourself with supportive people.

## Awareness and Advocacy

Scabies is a condition that needs more public education regarding its causes, symptoms, and available treatments. Outreach programs, educational initiatives, and calls for improved access to healthcare for scabies patients can help achieve this goal. More people learning about the illness means more people can understand and help those who live with it.

## Insights from Patients

It can be both enlightening and empowering to hear the tales of people who have lived with scabies. Successes, failures, and coping mechanisms in controlling the disease can be gleaned from these accounts. People coping with scabies often find hope and encouragement in hearing about the stories of others.

## Resources for Empowerment

Individuals impacted by scabies can find empowerment resources such as educational materials, self-help techniques, and access to support programs. Websites, booklets, hotlines, and support groups that offer information, encouragement, and practical advice for managing the disease effectively are examples of these resources.

## Fighting for What We Need

Scabies sufferers must keep their optimism and strength. Keep an optimistic outlook, pay attention to how far along you are in your treatment, and reach out for help when you need it. One way to overcome the difficulties of scabies and come out stronger is to have a resilient mindset.

People with scabies can improve their physical and emotional health and cope with the condition better if these areas are addressed thoroughly.